Basic P to

Note

This book describes a process that can be used to reduce stress or regulate intrapsychic processes and is also suitable as a self-help method. It has proven to be very effective and safe in practice. However, it cannot be ruled out, that its application by laymen can activate strong unwanted emotions, especially when traumatic memories are processed with it. The method described here is not a substitute for professional treatment.

Whoever processes his own concerns with this method does so in his own responsibility.

Michael Hoffmann

BASIC PEAT
to free your mind

Impressum

Bibliografische Information der Deutschen
Nationalbibliothek:
Die Deutsche Nationalbibliothek verzeichnet
diese Publikation in der Deutschen National-
bibliografie; detaillierte bibliografische Daten
sind im Internet über http://dnb.dnb.de
abrufbar.

TWENTYSIX – Der Self-Publishing-Verlag
Eine Kooperation zwischen der Verlagsgruppe
Random House und BoD – Books on Demand

© 2017 Michael Hoffmann

Herstellung und Verlag:
BoD – Books on Demand, Norderstedt

ISBN: 9783740733940

Illustration: Monika Huber
Translation: Mathew Davis
Proofreading: Melanie McGhee

Content

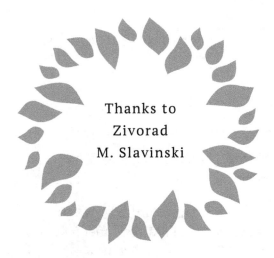

Thanks to
Zivorad
M. Slavinski

Acknowledgement

This book would not have come to existence without the direct or indirect support from some special people.

I would like to thank all of them for their personal contribution to the development of this book. My special thanks go to Zivorad M. Slavinski, my wife Renate, Monika Huber, Helmut Vizedum, Melanie McGhee, Mathew Davis and the participants in the Munich training group of PEAT and related methods.

Introduction

This booklet is an introduction to the Basic PEAT process of Zivorad M. Slavinski and is primarily intended as a practical guide for users. Basic PEAT (Primordial Energy Activation and Transcendence) is a very effective form of meridian therapy, which can be used both as a supplementary technique in the context of psychotherapeutic work and also as a self-help method for the elimination of mental and emotional stress.

The booklet is written in agreement and with the permission of Zivorad Slavinski and is kept as short as possible, especially in the theoretical part, because Zivorad Slavinski has already described the theory in detail in his own books. If you would like to know more about the theoretical background of PEAT, please refer to Slavinski's books. At the end of this booklet, you will find the relevant literature references.

If you want to study PEAT in a workshop, you can do so with any certified PEAT trainer. You can find a trainer on

http://spiritual-technology.com/?page_id=532

I. PEAT AND OTHER METHODS OF MERIDIAN TAPPING THERAPY

Basic PEAT (= Primordial Energy Activation and Transcendence) is a method which belongs to the field of »energy psychology« and is very well suited to mitigate or even eliminate, internal psychological stress of all kinds. PEAT can be applied both as a self-help method and in working with others.

The term »energy psychology« goes back to the American psychotherapist Roger J. Callahan, who in the late 1970s, began to combine elements of clinical psychology, traditional Chinese medicine and applied kinesiology, to develop his so-called »Thought Field Therapy« (TFT).

Callahan assumed that the body of a human being is traversed by a great number of energy channels – the so-called meridians –, each of which is connected to both, a bodily organ and a certain point on the body surface. His hypothesis was that diseases, pain and emotional and psychological problems may arise because the flow of energy in one of these meridians is blocked by a traumatic experience. If this was the case and one succeeded in freeing the flow of energy in the blocked meridian, the corresponding problems would then disappear. Callahan hoped that this liberation of the energy flow would be achieved by rhythmically tapping and thus activating a certain meridian point, while deliberately reminding oneself of the traumatic experience.

Thus, he developed the Thought Field Therapy,

where the user can tap a certain sequence of meridian points, while inwardly experiencing a problem that he wants to eliminate. This tapping of body points resulted in his method and those of his successor's, being called »tapping therapy«, »meridian therapy« and »tapping«.

Whether this hypothesis is true or not, the fact is that his method achieves astonishingly rapid and good results in the elimination of phobias and other emotional problems, which are now also confirmed by large-scale scientific studies (see below in the text). Callahan subsequently published several books on the application of TFT and expanded his knowledge.

In the period thereafter, other authors, inspired by Callahan's success, developed altered variants of tapping therapy or related self-creations based on the same principles as of TFT, but differing more or less, in their treatment processes from that of Callahan's.

Common among all is the assumption that the meridian or bio-energetic system of man plays a decisive role in the development and solution of emotional and psychological problems.

In all the processes, acupuncture points are stimulated by holding or tapping during the treatment of the problems.

While working on the problem, one has to focus on it. However, it should be formulated as specifically as possible. Complex problems should be divided into various components and then processed individually. For this, an experienced user or therapist can be helpful.

In the meantime, there are a growing number of energetic methods that can be attributed to the field of tapping therapy.

Some of them, well known in Germany, are:

1. **Thought Field Therapy (TFT)**
   by Roger J. Callahan (published around 1985)

2. **Emotional Freedom Techniques (EFT)**
   by Gary Craig (developed in the early nineties)

3. **Negative Affect Erasing Method (NAEM)**
   by Fred P. Gallo (developed around 1995)

4. **Emotional Self-Management (ESM)**
   by George Pratt and Peter Lambrou (published around 2000)

5. **Meridian Energy Technic (MET)**
   by Rainer Franke (developed around 2004)

6. **Process- and Embodiment-focused Psychology (PEP)** by Michael Bohne (published around 2006)

In addition, there are still some less known variants of tapping, as well as various energetic-psychological methods that combine elements of tapping with elements from NLP or other alternative therapies.

One of these less well-known methods (or groups of methods) is the so-called Primordial Energy Activation and Transcendence (PEAT) by Zivorad M. Slavinski, which was developed between 1999 and 2003 and is discussed in this booklet.

Regarding the efficacy of the tapping methods in general, numerous studies have been carried out over the last decades, the results of which were so encouraging that in 2012 they were finally approved by the American Psychological Association APA (the largest psychological association of the World) as an empirical field based therapy (= based on empirical field research).

Probably the most extensive of all these studies was conducted by Dr. Joaquin Andrade and based on data collected by 36 therapists in 11 clinics in Argentina and Uruguay over a period of 14 years on over 29,000 patients. Within the framework of this study, numerous studies with comparative groups were also carried out, for example, a five-and-a-half-year study on 5,000 patients with anxiety disorders. Half of the test subjects were treated with a tapping treatment and the other half, the control group, was treated with behavioral therapy and medication support, if applicable. The results showed that meridian therapy was more effective than behavioral therapy, and it also took less time.

Comparison: 5,000 patients with anxiety disorders at the end of therapy		
	Slight-improvement	Complete-recovery
Behaviourtherapy / medicines	63 %	51 %
Psychological energytreatment	90 %	76 %

As for the effectiveness of Basic PEAT, I found only one study on the Internet. This was done by Professor John Fitch, Joel DiGirolamo, and Laura Schmuldt at the Eastern Kentucky University in 2011 and published under the title »The Efficacy of PEAT to address public speaking anxiety« in the Journal Energy Psychology 3, 2, November 2011.

In this study, Fitch and his colleagues examined the impact of the application of the Basic PEAT process on anxiety. The study included 82 students who were divided into an experimental group and a control group. The participants had to prepare themselves for a speech that they had to hold in front of a large audience and their stress level was measured at different times. However, the participants of the experimental group also completed a 20 minute Basic PEAT process for stress reduction before the performance, while the participants of the control group did not. The result was that the experimental group showed a significantly lower level of anxiety immediately before and during the stage performance.

This study provides an indication that Basic PEAT, as far as efficacy is concerned, can be compared with EFT and other tapping methods.

II. SIMILARITIES AND DIFFERENCES BETWEEN BASIC PEAT AND OTHER METHODS OF MERIDIAN TAPPING THERAPY

But what is so special about PEAT, that it is worthwhile to engage with it?

Well, each of the existing PEAT variants has certain characteristics and peculiarities that make it attractive for therapists and users of self-help techniques. Common among all the variants is:

- that they are very easy to learn and can be applied by almost every person

- that the application takes very little time (often only 5 to 10 minutes)

- that they are very effective

- that they follow a holistic approach, thereby achieving more stable results and as a by-product of the application, lead to the strengthening of one's own empathy

- that they end with positive emotions.

The deep PEAT processes also show some special features, which are described in the last chapter of this booklet.

However, the following chapters are devoted to a detailed presentation of the Basic PEAT process, since among all PEAT variants, this has the most similarity to the already existing meridian tapping therapies. In addition, you will find a step by step guide of the Basic PEAT process, which you can try out yourself.

If you want to learn more about the deep PEAT processes after reading this booklet, you can refer to Zivorad Slivinski's books »PEAT - New Pathways«, »Transcendence« and »Return to Oneness«. Currently (in 2017), these books are available as e-books on http://www.arelena.com.

Let us now have a look at the similarities and differences between the Basic PEAT process and other methods of tapping.

Areas of application

The application areas for Basic PEAT are the same as for the other tapping methods as well. To summarize, these are usually the unwanted psychological and emotional states, negative thoughts and beliefs, unpleasant physical sensations, and crushing decisions that we have once made and which have a significant influence on our present life.

Basic PEAT is particularly suitable for the treatment of acute emotional stress, which builds up for example in daily work contexts. It is also suitable to address anger that builds up towards other people or certain situations, frustrations of any kind, jealousy, hatred, envy, revenge, feelings of overwhelm anxiety, phobias, worries, guilt feelings, embarrassment, sadness etc.

However, one has to be careful when dealing with severe traumatic experiences. A specialist should be sought in this case, or in case of any other serious psychological problems.

According to Zivorad Slavinski Basic PEAT has also proven to be effective in working with skin problems, muscle pains and tendon pains, back pain, neck pain, etc.

The bifocal approach

In all tapping and meridian therapies, negative, restrictive and stressful feelings are treated by tapping or holding certain points on the face, body and hands. This is where the popular term »tapping therapies« comes from.

Self-boycotting thoughts and restrictive beliefs, on the other hand, are treated with the help of so-called »self-acceptance sentences«.

This is also the case with Basic PEAT. In this, the meridian points are gently touched with the index finger and the middle finger, and the touch is held as long as it is required for a deep inhalation and exhalation. Self-acceptance sentences are used at the same time, and they always have the same structure as follows: »Even if I have this problem, I love and accept myself, my body, my personality, and the fact that I have this problem.« Thereby the specific problem is named each time.

The use of meridian points

In all the acupressure and meridian therapies, different acupressure points are stimulated. The number, sequence, and selection of acupressure points vary from method to method, ranging from a few to about 17 different points. In some meridian techniques, the order of the acupressure points to be stimulated is always the same, as per the Thought Field Therapy of Roger J. Callahan or the Emotional Self-Management of Lambrou and Pratt, wherein, one has to tap a specific sequence of points for each problem topic.

In Basic PEAT we only use 4 points: a point at the middle of the sternum and 3 points around the two eyes. The order of the touch is the same for every problem. This makes the Basic PEAT process easy for beginners, since 3 points can be easier memorized than 17, and the repetition is quickly automated.

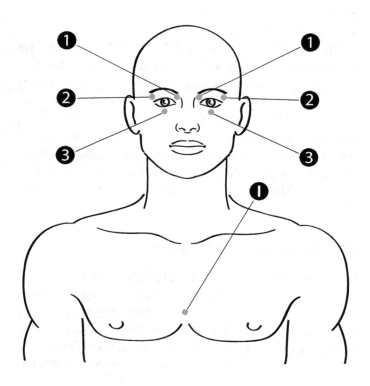

The assessment of the intensity of the perceived problem

In Basic PEAT, the focus is first drawn to the strength of the undesirable condition (0 = no problem noticeable, 5 = moderate problem intensity, 10 = the problem intensity is almost intolerable). This is an element that is also found in other meridian therapy systems. After the process, the strength of the problem should be zero because it will then no longer exist. The PEAT process is over, when the problem can no longer be felt as a problem. On an average, a process takes 15 minutes, which is often sufficient to eliminate the problem.

Deep breathing

Deep inhalation and exhalation is an element of the Basic PEAT process, which is not found in other meridian techniques.

However, since breathing energizes our whole body and its energy field, deep breathing supports the elimination of blocks in our energy. In addition, deep breathing helps to experience and release emotions as completely as possible, so that as far as possible, no suppressed residues are left over during processing.

Visualizing the problem as a snapshot

The stopping, reversing, slowing or accelerating of mental problem movie have long been elements of some NLP techniques (NLP = neuro linguistic programming), and have proved to be very helpful in dealing with phobias and other problems. However, this procedure is not common in conventional tapping methods.

During the Basic PEAT process, the three points around both eyes are alternately touched, while one focusses on the worst moment of an experience. For this, one has to stop the inner problem movie at its most dramatic moment, turn it into a snapshot and make sure that the picture does not return into a movie again.

Stopping in time, prevents the problem film from being repeated in the same or a roughly modified form again. This way of mentally going through a problem repeatedly, however, is necessary and responsible for the maintenance of any problem.

So the conversion of the problem movie into a snapshot accelerates the process of its resolution.

However, it is also possible to use Basic PEAT with bad feelings in one's current experience without necessarily creating a snapshot (for example »I'm feeling stressed because ...«). Here one works with the general feeling of stress.

Considering the future

There are already other self-help methods, in which it is examined whether the client believes that his problem can arise again in the future. But this is still rarely the case with standard meridian techniques. This is a deficit that is taken into consideration in the Basic PEAT process. Experience shows that even if clients can not feel their initial problem at the end of the process anymore, many of them nevertheless doubt that this outcome will be lasting. This means, however, that there is still some emotional charge related to the problem that needs to be eliminated.

In Basic PEAT, the future is examined with the question »Do you think that your problem will return to you against your will in the future?« If the client agrees to this question, he is asked to visualize this scenario and we perform a Basic PEAT process on it: »Feel that your problem returns to you in the future, against your will. Feel this as intensively as you can and create the appropriate inner vision of how this happens. Then stop this vision at its worst moment, make a snapshot of it and ...« (apply the process)

Circular processing of the problem

The consideration of other points of view in the processing of problems is an element which is applied in many psycho-energetic methods of Zivorad Slavinski. As far as I know, no other method of meridian acupuncture tapping is using it until now.

Since in Basic PEAT we follow a holistic approach, problems must be solved from all important points of view.

While Zivorad Slavinski explains the value of circular processing from a metaphysical perspective, I would like to focus on a simple psychological aspect.

If we are suffering from an interpersonal problem, we automatically assume that our adversaries are holding certain intentions, attitudes and thoughts. We suspect their actions to be inconsiderate, malicious or reckless; think that they are incapable or are suffering from weakness in character etc. These assumptions can be more or less correct, but also completely false. But whether they are right or not, they have a huge impact on our perception of the problem.

Thereby, we usually take our own standpoints for

granted, we don't question them, and overlook or deny that other's viewpoints may also contain a grain of truth, that they may be justified, and that the others may feel different from what we suppose.

We focus our attention only on one half of the entire experience, ignoring the other half and pretending as if it didn't exist. However, the holistic approach also takes into account the other side of the experience, which is usually dispelled in the shadow.

If one removes only one's own concern during the problem treatment, this shadow unfortunately remains. One can thus continue to cheat around it and build up a new negative emotional charge. The problem then is not completely eliminated, and an important aspect of it persists. Apart from this, in this case, one never assumes full responsibility for one's own actions.

Two examples:

CASE STUDY 1

A 16-year-old client had a conflict with a roommate of his residential community and asked for help because he was about to start a fight with him. We first worked on his anger, which disappeared after about 10 minutes. This surprised him deeply. Then I asked him to do the process from his roommate's perspective too. At first, he was reluctant, but then agreed to do so out of curiosity. This process too was done quickly and the young man began to grin. To my question »what was going on?«, he replied that he probably would had reacted the same way as his roommate and that now, I have spoiled his fun of feeling superior to the other.

CASE STUDY 2

The mother of a client was dying and the client wanted to apply a PEAT process to the problem, as he could not behave naturally in front of his mother because he was emotionally overwhelmed by the situation. He felt uncomfortable and insecure in her presence, so he avoided contact with her, and that made him feel guilty. The process was easy and the client reported after less than 20 minutes, that he could now imagine feeling comfortable in his mother's presence. Then we did the process from the perspective of all people involved in the problem. These were essentially his sick mother, his siblings and his father. Both the sibling's and mother's positions had little emotional impact, but when he took the position of his father, he was flooded by a deep mourning and despair that caught him by surprise. After processing from the father's position, he could face his mother calmly again, and he had also gained a completely new understanding for his father.

Filling with light

Filling with light is a typical component of many of the psycho-energetic methods developed by Zivorad Slavinski, which is not found in other meridian techniques.

Since at the end of a successful PEAT process a kind of vacuum exists at the place where the problem had previously been felt, we fill light into it. If this is not done, there is a risk that the vacuum will suck up the problem again, or attract other negative content that is similar to the problem that has been solved. To avoid this, in other methods a positive state is installed, which can also be done after the Basic PEAT process.

Light is particularly suitable for filling emptiness as it is neutral by itself. However, as a source of all life, light has a soothing effect on our body and mind.

Forgiveness

In his book »PEAT – new pathways« Zivorad Slavinski writes: »Until recently, the fields of psychiatry and psychology seldom if ever mentioned forgiveness ... However, practical therapeutic experience shows that forgiveness can be very critical to prolonging the effects of a therapeutic process.«

If we cannot forgive ourselves or the persons who contributed to our problem at the end of a PEAT process, this means that there is still some energy in the problem. But no matter how little energy is left in it, sooner or later it may undermine a process that would have otherwise been successful and cause the problem to return.

To avoid this, in Basic PEAT a forgiveness exercise is included. When the procedure of forgiving is done, a deep harmony with oneself and the world is attained and the results of the therapeutic work are more stable.

III. HOW PEAT WAS DEVELOPED

Though this manual is dedicated to Basic PEAT, it will be helpful to understand the history of this pioneering methodology. All PEAT processes originate from the creative work of the clinical psychologist Zivorad M. Slavinski, who created several highly effective psycho-energetic healing systems during the 1980s and 1990s. When Slavinski developed the deep PEAT process during the course of his research and experiments in 1999, he was deeply impressed by its effects from the outset.

PEAT stands for Primordial Energy Activation and Transcendence. According to Slavinski, with this method it is possible to integrate the deepest inner conflict of a human being, whereby the energy, which is bound by it, is set free and is used for transcendence. By the application of deep PEAT this deepest inner conflict, which is the basis of our inner turmoil and thus the basis of our drama of life, can be made conscious, energetically discharged and thus solved as a problem. During this process a lot of psychic energy is set free, which allows us to experience the space beyond the opposites for a short time.

After years of research and experimentation, deep PEAT became as easy and fast as it is today. In the early days, Deep PEAT could take up to three hours. Now, with added refinements, the core sequence of the deep PEAT process often does not take more than 10 to 25 minutes.

Slavinski is fond of saying »simplicity is close to perfection.« The development of his elegant methods demonstrates this axiom. Slavinski continued experimenting and looking for a simpler and faster version of Deep PEAT. Through diligent practice and study of his results, Slavinski developed the Basic PEAT process in 2000. The newly discovered process could be carried out much more quickly, but was less profound than the deep PEAT process. He initially named it Shallow PEAT, but later changed the name to Basic PEAT after some optimization. By embedding it into a holistic approach typical of Slavinski's methods (see also »checking the future« and »circular processing«), the effectiveness and sustainability of the results could finally be significantly increased. Thus, Basic PEAT became an excellent instrument of rapid self-regulation and valuable therapeutic technology. While many other methods developed by Slavinski have the capacity to find and eliminate the deepest inner conflicts of a person, Basic PEAT is a »go-to« tool for clients and others committed to cultivating a steadier inner state.

After the development of the Basic PEAT process, Zivorad Slavinski continued his search for similar techniques. Over the course of the following years, three further variants of the deep PEAT process (also called DP-2, DP-3 and DP-4) were developed. Each of them has its own special qualities, which are described in the last chapter of this booklet.

IV. PRELIMINARY EXERCISES

When you perform the Basic PEAT process for the first time, it is useful to perform some acceptance exercises as well as 2 to 3 snapshot exercises. Though this is not absolutely necessary, it gives a better understanding of what an attitude of acceptance really means and how to create visualized snapshots. For the success of the PEAT process, it is crucial to consider the selected problem experience as a snapshot during processing. Additionally, one should not allow any resistance towards it and thus for a short time, accept the unpleasant feeling.

Apart from this, you should briefly familiarize yourself with the process, so that you know what is going to happen.

Acceptance Exercises

Look around the room you are in and find an object that you like. Now accept this object and the fact that you like it, by thinking: »Yes, I accept this object and I like it.«

Now look for something that you do not like and accept this too: »Yes, I accept this object and I do not like it.«

Now close your eyes and recall some nice moments from the past. Watch the mental movie of this moment and accept it by saying, »Yes, I accept this memory.«

Now keep your eyes closed and recall some unpleasant experience. Watch the mental movie of this moment and accept it by saying, »Yes, I accept this memory.«

Finally recall some experience and feel yourself to be right in the middle of the experience, as if it were happening right now. Accept it without any resistance. Now accept the different elements of this memory one by one: the image of the experience, the emotion that you feel in this experience, the body sensation and the thoughts that you have.

Snapshot Exercise

Close your eyes and remember a problematic situation. Now, choose that moment of this situation, which to you seems to be the most dramatic or unpleasant. Stop the memory at this most dramatic moment, as if you were pressing a pause button on a video player. This gives you a still image in which no movement or change takes place anymore.

V. BASIC PEAT: THE PROCESS

Basic PEAT consists of the following 11 steps:

1. Define the problem that you want to solve, as specifically as possible

2. Define, how you want to feel in such a situation in the future

3. Touch the chest point and pronounce the self-acceptance phrase

4. Feel your problem and estimate its intensity on a scale of 0 to 10

5. Perform the Basic PEAT core process until the intensity of the problem is zero

6. Review the results

7. Consider the future

8. Circular processing

9. Forgiveness

10. Filling with light

11. Installation of a positive attitude

Step 1
Define the problem (that) you want to solve

In the beginning you must first define the problem that you want to solve. If you are working with another person, let her/him briefly describe the problem. This should not take more than a few minutes. The problem formulation should be as specific as possible and should have the following structure: »I feel ... about ...«

Examples of specific problems:

»I'm afraid of spiders« (= I feel scared of spiders)
»I hate my neighbor« (= I feel hatred towards my neighbor)

Unspecific problems can be eliminated in the short term, but they tend to return. Therefore, they should be avoided.

Examples of unspecific problems:

»It's all too much for me«
»I am depressed!«

Unspecific problems should be broken down into their various components, which are then to be processed individually. In the examples just given, you could ask the client, what exactly leads him to this experience. After noting down the different situations and the associated emotions, which the client describes, you can then process them one by one.

Step 2
Define the goal of the session

After you have defined the problem according to the above structure »I feel ... about ...«, consider briefly what you want to feel instead, or how you want to be able deal with the problem situation in the future. Keep in mind that you can only change your own responses to the unwanted situations, but not the circumstances themselves.

Examples of suitable goals:

»I want to be relaxed in front of spiders. «
»I want to be able to stay cool, when I meet my neighbor. «

Examples of unsuitable goals:

»I never want to meet a spider again.«
»I want my neighbor to move away.«

Step 3
Touch your chest point and say the self-acceptance sentence loud

Now touch your chest point (at the center of your sternum) gently with the index finger and middle finger of one of your hands (doesn't matter which one), and pronounce the self-acceptance phrase to resolve any self-sabotage tendencies. The self-acceptance phrase has the same structure for each problem and is:

»*Even though ... I love and accept myself, my body, my personality and the fact, that ...*«
Instead of the dots, the respective problem should be mentioned.

In the examples just described, this would look like this:

»Even though I am afraid of spiders, I love and accept myself, my body, my personality and the fact, that I am afraid of spiders.«

»Even though I hate my neighbor, I love and accept myself, my body, my personality and the fact, that I hate my neighbor.«

Step 4
Feel the problem as completely as possible and estimate its strength

Close your eyes and visualize your problem. Feel your problem and pay attention to your memory film. As you walk through the scene, stop the movie at its most dramatic moment, so that you get a still image.

Now estimate the intensity of the perceived problem on a scale of 0 to 10 (0 = no problem, 10 = intolerable problem).

Step 5
Perform the Basic PEAT core process until the intensity of the problem is at zero.

In the course of the process, be sure to focus on this still image of the most dramatic moment and be careful that the memory does not change into a movie again.

Look at the »frozen« image of the most dramatic moment of the problem situation the way you saw it then. Feel what you felt then, think what you thought then. The more deep you slip into this experience, the faster the emotional charge will dissolve.

Now touch the following points in sequence, while your attention is fully focused on the problem. Deeply inhale and exhale at the end of each touch. Unlike other meridian therapies, there is no need to tap; a light touch is all that is needed.

THE BASIS PEAT CORE PROCESS:

1. Left side, first eye point (with left hand) –
      inhale and exhale deeply
   Right side, first eye point (with right hand) –
      inhale and exhale deeply

2. Left side, second eye point (with left hand) –
      inhale and exhale deeply
   Right side, second eye point (with right hand) -
      inhale and exhale deeply

3. Left side, third eye point (with left hand) –
      inhale and exhale deeply
   Right side, third eye point (with right hand) -
      inhale and exhale deeply

After you have gone through all 6 eye points, estimate the intensity of the problem again on a scale of 0 to 10 (0 = no problem at all, 10 = intolerable problem). The problem should now be much weaker or should have even completely disappeared. If the problem strength has not yet arrived at 0, repeat the sequence from point 3 until you can no longer feel the problem. On an average, you will need 3 to 5 repetitions for this. Adjust the self-acceptance phrase to your actual feelings.

Example:
»Even though I can still feel a bit of my fear of spiders, I love and accept myself, my body, my personality, and the fact that I can still feel a bit of my fear of spiders.«

Now touch the 6 eye points one by one while your attention is fully focused on the problem and breathe deeply in and out at the end of each touch.

1. Left side, first eye point (with left hand) –
        inhale and exhale deeply
    Right side, first eye point (with right hand) –
        inhale and exhale deeply

2. Left side, second eye point (with left hand) –
        inhale and exhale deeply
    Right side, second eye point (with right hand) -
        inhale and exhale deeply

3. Left side, third eye point (with left hand) –
        inhale and exhale deeply
    Right side, third eye point (with right hand) -
        inhale and exhale deeply

Repeat this sequence until the problem has completely disappeared.

Step 6
Check the result

Now, to check the result, ask yourself what has happened to the problem: »*What has happened to the problem ... (name it)? Do I still feel it as a problem or not?*«

If you still feel it as a problem, re-estimate the

strength of the problem and restart with step 5 (the Basic PEAT core process).

If your problem has disappeared, continue with step 7.

Step 7
Check the future

To check whether you have unconscious objections to the healing of your problem, which would result in the problem returning, ask yourself whether you currently believe or feel that your problem can come back to you in the future **against your will** or not. (The emphasis should be on »**against your will**«)

If »not« move to step 8.

If »yes«, please speak the self-acceptance phrase:

»*Even though I believe or think that my problem* (name the problem) *may reappear **against my will** in the future, I love and accept myself, my body, my personality and the fact that I believe or think my problem may reappear in the future **against my will**.*«

Then imagine a future situation in which the problem will reappear against your will, make a snapshot of the most dramatic moment in your mind's eye and enter into this situation as if it were happening now. Then check the strength of the problem which you feel has returned to you and do a Basic PEAT core process on it (step 5 to step 6).

Continue with it until you make sure, that the problem will not come back to you against your will anymore and you no longer worry about the future re-emergence of the problem.

When you have reached the point where you have completely discharged your problem, you will likely feel a sense of relief and clarity that you can choose to react differently to the same or similar situations in the future.

If no other person or living being is involved in your problem, you can skip step 8 and complete the process with step 9.

If, however, other people or creatures are involved in your problem, proceed with circular processing in step 8.

Step 8
Apply the Basic PEAT process also from the perspectives of all other persons or living beings involved in the problem (= circular processing)

Ask yourself if other people or creatures are involved in your problem. If so, in your imagination, take the perspective of the persons (or creatures) involved (one by one), feel like that person (or creature) feels, think how that person (or creature) thinks, see and experience what that person (or creature) sees and experiences.

Referring to the examples from before, namely the fear of spiders and the hatred towards the neighbor, the circular processes would look like the following:

Working on the fear of spiders:
Close your eyes and touch your chest with your index finger and middle finger, and say, *»I am no longer ... (say your name), but a spider. «*

Then, in your imagination, you should identify with

the perspective of a spider as far as possible. Be a spider. Then ask yourself how you feel as a spider when you hear that ... (add your name at this point) is afraid of you as a spider. If you have an emotional response as a reaction to this question, perform a complete Basic PEAT process, starting with the self-acceptance phrase at step 3 and ending with step 6. (Checking the future is not necessary in circular processing) Stay in the perspective of a spider during the whole process.

When all emotional charge has disappeared, touch your chest with the index finger and middle finger, and say the following sentence: »*I am not a spider anymore. I am ... (say your name) again.*«

Then move to step 9.

Working on the hatred towards your neighbor:

Close your eyes and touch your chest with your index finger and middle finger, and say the following sentence: »*I am no longer ... (say your name), but mister ... (tell the name of your neighbor).* «

Then, in your imagination, enter into your neighbor's perspective as completely as possible. Be your neighbor. Think like your neighbor. Feel like your neighbor. Then ask yourself as you would ask your neighbor, how you feel when you hear that ... (insert your name at this point) hates you. If you have an emotional response to this question, perform a complete Basic PEAT process, starting with the self-acceptance phrase at step 3 and ending with step 6. (Checking the future is not necessary in circular processing) Stay in the perspective of your neighbor during the whole process.

When all emotional charge has disappeared, touch your chest with the index finger and middle finger, and speak the following sentence: »*I am not Mr* ... (neighbor's name) *anymore, but again* ... (say your name). «

Check if other people are involved in or are affected by your hatred towards your neighbor. If so, do Basic PEAT processes from the perspective of everyone involved. If not, move on to step 9.

Step 9
Forgiveness

In order to remove the last vestiges of negative emotional charge, we continue with a forgiveness exercise. For this, place two fingers on your chest point and say the following, while really feeling the words:

»*I forgive God* (cosmic force, universe, or whatever you believe in) *for creating this world in which some people suffer from* (insert your problem – fear of spiders; hatred towards neighbor). *I forgive all beings who contributed to the creation of this problem of mine and I forgive myself for creating and maintaining this problem.*«

Step 10
Fill yourself with light

Since the elimination of the negative state creates a kind of vacuum in the psyche, there is a risk that after the process you will activate a new unwanted content in the place where the problem was before. To prevent this, you should fill the vacuum with light at the end of the process.

»*Imagine a ball of bright white light hovering 20 cm above your head. While taking a deep breath in, imagine that a light beam from this light ball enters your head, neck and shoulders and fills the upper part of your body with light.* (pause) *Then breathe in a second time, imagining that you are drawing in more light and filling the lower part of your body with it.* (pause) *Inhale a third time, and imagine filling your arms and legs with the light.* (pause) *Now, draw even more light into yourself and let it spread around your body in the form of a radiant aura. Now see and feel this glowing aura for about 10 seconds and open your eyes again whenever you want.*«

Step 11
Install a positive attitude

To conclude, consider briefly how you want to react in the future to situations that you have experienced as a problem up until now.

In the above examples of the fear of spiders and hatred of your neighbor, serenity and tranquility could be good options to counter it. However, decide for yourself how you want to react towards them.

Then close your eyes and imagine yourself to be in the future, reacting in the desired way (for example, see yourself staying calm in the face of a spider or being indifferent in an encounter with your neighbor). In doing so, you should see yourself from the outside, as through a camera.

Then, touch the six points around your eyes in the reverse order and enter the positive scenario as fully as possible. (To take the earlier examples, feel as relaxed and calm as possible):

1. Right side, third eye point (with right hand) –
        inhale and exhale deeply
    Left side, third eye point (with left hand) –
        inhale and exhale deeply

2. Right side, second eye point (with right hand) –
        inhale and exhale deeply
    Left side, second eye point (with left hand) –
        inhale and exhale deeply

3. Right side, first eye point (with right hand) –
        inhale and exhale deeply
    Left side, first eye point (with left hand) –
        inhale and exhale deeply

When you can feel the positive reaction clearly, the
process is finished.

VI. IMPORTANT HINTS

1. The Basic PEAT process can only directly influence the way you evaluate a situation or an event and how you feel about it. It cannot however, directly change the circumstances or events themselves. This should be absolutely clear; otherwise you will have wrong expectations from the process and thereafter be disappointed. For this reason, you need to be careful not to choose PEAT to process situations and events, but to process your feeling towards them. The statements »I have lost my job« or »my wife has separated from me« are events. »I fear losing my livelihood because I've lost my job,« or »I'm desperate because my wife has left me,« are problems that can be handled with PEAT.

2. The problem to be worked on should always be described as specifically as possible! If the problem description is not specific (e.g., »I'm feeling bad«), it should be divided into the components, of which it is composed. These can then be processed individually.

3. During a Basic PEAT process you should release as much resistance as possible towards the experience you are working on. Since resistance is one of the main reasons for having problems at all, you should better switch to an attitude of curiosity,

readiness, or acceptance. This point is of crucial importance for successful processing. Remember, to accept something doesn't mean you have to approve of or like it.

4. Basic PEAT can be practiced alone or with a partner. Some people find it easier to work with a partner, since in this case one can concentrate on leading the process and the other can concentrate on following the instructions. When they are guided through the process, their attention doesn't get distracted so easily.

5. The application of Basic PEAT is not a substitute for necessary action. If for example, you are stuck in a harmful relationship or at a workplace, where conditions are detrimental to your own health, you can process the resulting emotional stress many times, only to get short-term relief from these processes. In such cases only a separation or change of job may help. You cannot escape the fact that you have to take action.

6. Although Basic PEAT is highly effective when dealing with emotional problems and other psychological stressors, it is not a substitute for medical help if one has serious mental problems. But even then, it can be a valuable supplement for any treatment. If you are experiencing unexpected psycho-emotional problems during the application of Basic PEAT or if the problems you are experiencing do not disappear, you should consult a specialist. As mentioned, caution is recommended when dealing with heavy trauma.

One last tip: TRY IT OUT! Reading alone is no good. As the saying goes: »If you want to know how a pudding tastes, you must eat it. Reading the recipe is not enough.«

VII. BASIC PEAT MANUAL
FOR THE APPLICATION TO OTHERS

1. *Please briefly describe your problem in a few words.* (Write down the answer)

2. *How would you prefer to feel in this situation or how would you prefer to approach this problem?* (Write down the answer)

3. *Now close your eyes, touch the chest point and say, »Even if I ...* (name the problem), *I love and accept myself, my body, my personality and the fact that I ...* (name the problem).«

4. *Now, remember your problem. Feel yourself in your problem and pay attention to the problem movie. As you go through the scene, stop the movie at the most dramatic moment, so that you see it as a snapshot. In the further course of the process, focus on this snapshot of the most dramatic moment, and make sure that the snapshot does not change into a movie again.*

    Rate the strength of your problem on a 10 point scale, where 10 is the maximum problem strength. (Write down the answer)

5 a) *Now touch the first eyepoint on the left, underneath the eyebrow, close to the bridge of the noise with the index and middle finger of your left hand. Fully absorb yourself into your negative*

experience, feel it completely and without internal resistance. See what you have seen in that moment. Hear what you heard in that moment. Feel this moment, not a second sooner and not a second later, as if it were happening now ... – Deeply inhale and exhale.

5 b) *Now, with the index and middle finger of your right hand touch the first eyepoint on the right side under the eyebrow close to the bridge of the nose. Fully absorb yourself into your negative experience, feel it completely and without internal resistance. See what you saw in that moment. Hear what you heard in that moment. Feel this moment, not a second sooner and not a second later, as if it were happening now ... – Deeply inhale and exhale.*

5 c) *Now touch the second eyepoint on the left side of the eye at the temple with the index and middle finger of the left hand.Fully absorb yourself into your negative experience, feel it completely and without internal resistance. See what you saw in that moment. Hear what you heard in that moment. Feel this moment, not a second sooner and not a second later, as if it were happening now ... – Deeply inhale and exhale.*

5 d) *With the index and middle finger of the right hand, touch the second eyepoint on the right side. Fully absorb yourself into your negative experience, feel it completely and without internal resistance. See what you saw in that moment. Hear what you heard in that moment. Feel this mo-*

ment, not a second sooner and not a second later, as if it were happening now ... – Deeply inhale and exhale.

5 e) *Now touch the point below your left eye with the index and middle finger of your left hand. Fully absorb yourself into your negative experience, feel it completely and without internal resistance. See what you saw in that moment. Hear what you heard in that moment. Feel this moment, not a second sooner and not a second later, as if it were happening now ... – Deeply inhale and exhale.*

5 f) *Now touch the point below your right eye with the index and middle finger of your right hand. Fully absorb yourself into your negative experience, feel it completely and without internal resistance. See what you saw in that moment. Hear what you heard in that moment. Feel this moment, not a second sooner and not a second later, as if it were happening now ... – Deeply inhale and exhale.*

6. *Estimate the intensity of your problem again on a scale of 0 to 10 (0 = no problem at all, 10 = intolerable problem).*

   (If the answer is 0, continue with step 6 a.) If the answer is not yet 0, ask your partner to speak an acceptance phrase: *»Even though I still feel my problem ...* (name the problem), *I love and accept myself, my body, my personality, and the fact that I still feel my problem ...* (name the problem).*«* Then continue with the Basic PEAT core process (step 5 a to 5 f) until the problem strength is at 0. Then proceed with 6 a.

6 a) *Now open your eyes and tell me what has happened to your problem ...* (name the problem)*? Do you still feel it as a problem or not?*

(The answer should be »no«.)

7. *Do you think that ...* (name the problem) *will be a problem for you against your will again in the future or not?*

(if »no«, continue with step 8. If »yes«, ask your client to speak an acceptance phrase):

»Even though I believe that my problem (name the problem) *may reappear against my will in the future, I love and accept myself, my body, my personality and the fact that I believe my problem may reappear in the future against my will «*

Imagine a future situation in which the problem comes back to you against your will, make a snapshot of the most dramatic moment in your mind's eye, and enter (into) this situation as if it were happening right now. Estimate the strength of the re-emerging problem.

(Now do another Basic PEAT process from step 5 a to 5 f, until the strength of the problem is 0.)

8. *Are there any other people involved in your problem?*

(If »no«, continue with step 11. If »yes«, ask for the names of these people, write them down and tell your client, to identify with each one of them. Apply a Basic PEAT process on the original problem from each of these person's perspectives.)

Close your eyes and touch your chest point with the index and middle finger, and speak the

following sentence: »I am not ... (fill in your own name) *any more, but ...* (fill in the name of the other person).«*
Imagine entering into the perspective of ... (fill in the name of the other person).
Be ... (fill in the name of the other person).
Think like ... (fill in the name of the other person*).*
Feel like ... (fill in the name of the other person).
As ..., how do you feel when you hear that ... (insert your name at this point) ... (name the problem)*?*

If you receive an emotional response to this question, perform a complete Basic PEAT process, starting with the self-acceptance phrase and ending with step 6a. Checking the future is not necessary for circular processing. Your partner should identify all the time with the other person and experience the corresponding perspective.

(When all emotional charge has disappeared):
Touch your chest point with the middle finger and repeat the following sentence: »I am no longer ... (name of the other person)*, but again ...«* (name of the client).

(Check if there are other people involved in the problem, and if so, perform PEAT processes from all of these perspectives, if not, go to step 9.)

9. *Do you feel a need to forgive or for forgiveness?* (if »no«, continue with step 10. If »yes«, ask your client if he believes in God, a cosmic force or any higher power. Then ask him to speak the forgiveness phrase):

   »I forgive God (cosmic force, universe, or whatever you believe in) for creating this world in which

some people suffer from ... (name the problem). *I forgive all beings who contributed to the creation of this problem of mine and I forgive myself for creating and maintaining this problem.*«

10. *Imagine a ball of bright white light hovering twenty centimeters above your head. Now take a deep breath and imagine that a light beam from this light ball enters your head, neck and chest area and fills the upper part of your body with light.* (pause) *Then take another deep breath and imagine that even more light is entering you and filling the lower part of your body.* (pause) *Then deeply inhale a third time and imagine that your arms and legs are filled with the light.* (pause) *Now take a fourth deep breath, draw even more light into your body and even spread it around your body in the form of a radiant aura. Look and feel this glowing aura for about 10 seconds.* (Now give the client some time.)

11. *How would you like to react in the future in situations similar to the problem situation?*
    (let the client answer).
    Close your eyes and imagine yourself in the future, experiencing the problematic situation. But now, see yourself reacting in the desired way, feeling the desired emotion and attitude (name it). *Watch this vision as seen through the eyes of another.*

11 a) *Now touch the point below your right eye with the index and middle finger of your right hand. Visualize the future event and how you master it*

in the desired way. See yourself from outside as you show the desired behavior and feel the desired emotion as strongly as possible ... as if it's happening now ... – Deeply inhale and exhale.

11 b) *Now touch the point below your left eye with the index and middle finger of your left hand. Visualize the future event and how you master it in the desired way. See yourself from outside as you show the desired behavior and feel the desired emotion as strongly as possible ... – Deeply inhale and exhale.*

11 c) *Now touch the point to the right of your right eye with the index and middle finger of your right hand. Visualize the future event and how you master it in the desired way. See yourself from outside as you show the desired behavior and feel the desired emotion as strongly as possible ... – Deeply inhale and exhale.*

11 d) *Now touch the point to the left of your left eye with the index and middle finger of your left hand. Visualize the future event and how you master it in the desired way. See yourself from outside as you show the desired behavior and feel the desired emotion as strongly as possible ... – Deeply inhale and exhale.*

11 e) *Now, with the index and middle finger of your right hand touch the eyepoint on the right side under the eyebrow close to the bridge of the nose. Visualize the future event and how you master it in the desired way. See yourself as you show the*

desired behavior and feel the desired emotion as strongly as possible ... – Deeply inhale and exhale.

11 f) *Now touch the first eyepoint on the left, underneath the eyebrow, close to the bridge of the nose with the index and middle finger of your left hand. Visualize the future event and how you master it in the desired way. See yourself as you show the desired behavior and feel the desired emotion as strongly as possible ... – Deeply inhale and exhale.*

Do you feel that you can react in a future situation of this kind as you have just imagined? (The clients answer should be »yes« at this point)

VIII. THE APPLICATION OF BASIS PEAT
TO PHYSICAL PROBLEMS

Basic PEAT is essentially a method of emotional self-regulation and elimination of mental stress. I use it almost exclusively for this purpose.

However, I know from Zivorad Slavinski that he also got good results in dealing with psychosomatic problems and pain. For this reason, I would like to give you an indication of how to proceed in these cases.

Treat the moment, when the problem appeared for the first time:

1. Briefly focus on your physical problem or pain and remember the moment when this problem or pain first occurred.

2. Stop the mental movie of this memory at its most dramatic moment and create a snapshot of that moment.

3. Step into this snapshot, experience it as fully as possible, and rate the problem on a 10 point scale.

4. Then, run the full Basic PEAT process until the problem has either disappeared or at least significantly weakened.

If the physical problem or the pain does not disappear,

you can at least treat your psychological reactions towards it.

Treat your inner responses to the physical problem:

1. Focus briefly on your physical problem or your pain.

2. Write down all the emotions or beliefs that appear within you towards this problem.

3. Then perform a Basic PEAT process on each emotion and belief.

Examples:

- Resistance to pain or non-acceptance of pain

- Grief because the body ages

- Anger because the body betrays you

- Protest because the body does not serve you the way you want it

- Criticism of parents who have predispositions against you

- Criticism of physicians who have not been able to help you

- Fear that you may never get well again.

- Fear of being handicapped in daily life

Process your physical problem from the point of view of your body (= circular processing):

For this, in your imagination, take the perspective of your physical body and feel, think and experience as your body might feel, think and experience about your physical problem. Then apply Basic PEAT on these contents.

IX. INTRODUCTION INTO THE VARIOUS FORMS OF DEEP PEAT

As already mentioned, the Basic PEAT process is only one of 4 PEAT variants currently being taught. In addition to Basic PEAT, there are also 3 different versions of the deep PEAT process, which for practical reasons are simply called Deep PEAT, DP-2 (Deep PEAT 2) and DP-4 (Deep PEAT 4). Each one of them has their respective advantages and disadvantages and / or application possibilities. Previously, there was also a DP-3 variant, which however was replaced by the DP-4 variant due to the higher efficiency of the later one.

The term »primordial energy activation and transcendence« (PEAT) is related to the fact that the deep PEAT process can be used to identify and integrate the primordial polarities of a human being, which is the basis of his life's drama. It is made conscious, discharged energetically and thus solved as a problem.

The term *primordial* refers to precisely this polarity in the life of a human being, which is the source of all her/his inner turmoil. *Primordial Energy Activation*, in turn, refers to the fact that in this polarity, a large amount of emotional and mental energy is bound, which is released by integration and is available to the individual again. The term *transcendence* refers to the fact that, at the moment of integration, one goes beyond polarities and thus transcends them.

Deep PEAT, mentioned earlier, is not simply a pure tapping technique. Deep PEAT is a holistic approach that includes elements of polarity integration and other aspects typical of Slavinski's methods. As a psychologist practicing since more than 15 years, I can say with confidence that the deep PEAT process is currently the most powerful weapon in the fight against the negative side effects of duality that exists at the moment. For this reason, American professor John Fitch from Eastern Kentucky University even referred to Deep PEAT as »EFT on steroids«.

Deep PEAT is the most complex and elaborate of the PEAT techniques and has some similarities to Basic PEAT. In Deep PEAT we use a combination of deep breathing, touching different acupuncture points and speaking acceptance phrases to reach into deeper layers of the chosen problem down to its origin. Then we identify the two poles of this problem source, which together form the primordial polarity of human beings. The two poles are then integrated. Since this primordial polarity is of particular importance and extreme value to the life of a person, the effect of its integration is often very intense and can have life-changing consequences. On the one hand, we experience the deepest non-dual state, which is available for us at the time of the integration, and on the other hand the problem that was connected with the primordial polarity disappears forever for most users.

DP-2 Is the abbreviation for Deep PEAT Level 2. With DP-2, emotional problems can be discharged in a short time by switching between emotional and cognitive contents with an accepting attitude. DP-2 is particularly effective in people who tend to intellectualize and have difficulty to feel something. It often lasts no longer than 15 minutes.

DP-4 (= Deep PEAT Level 4) is a method of polarity integration, during which one stimulates the first eye points of both eyes by touching them. The DP-4 process is a faster version of its predecessor DP-3, which is why the latter has been completely replaced. DP-4 doesn't go as deep as Deep PEAT, but has numerous applications and is easier and faster to run. A DP-4 process takes only 15 minutes and leads to polarity integration with almost every application. With DP-4, emotional and mental problems can be permanently eliminated in record speed. In addition, it is also possible to integrate specifically formulated polarities at the same rate and to integrate desired personality traits into one's own personality. DP-4 can also be used to integrate the shadow. DP-4 is not suitable to deal with highly complex problems such as addictions or personality disorders, in one step. These kinds of problems have to be broken into their components and these have to be processed one by one.

Deep PEAT

Let us return to the deep PEAT process, which many users refer to as a quantum leap in its area, because of both, its therapeutic and spiritual effectiveness. Even people like Tony Robbins, one of the most successful motivational and mental coaches in the world, are among the current fans of Deep PEAT.

This is not a surprise for two reasons. Firstly, with Deep PEAT, sometimes it is possible to solve even severe emotional and psychological problems in less than half an hour. Secondly, Deep PEAT is one of the very few publicly accessible processes which have the capacity to discover and integrate a person's primordial polarity, which is the root of most of his fundamental problems. Other terms for primordial polarity which can be found on the Internet, are »personal code« or »primes«.

But what is this primordial polarity? Its two poles represent the most fundamental pair of »approach or avoid« themes in our lives, which exert a compelling force on us. Thereby, no side is perceived exclusively as positive or negative. Rather, the dynamics resemble the principle of alternating current, in which each pole is alternately positively and negatively polarized. So, at a certain time in life we feel magically attracted by the one pole of the primordial polarity and do everything to reach it. But when we draw close to this pole to a certain point, the attraction changes and we suddenly feel drawn to the opposite pole with equal force. A widespread example of this phenomenon is the conflict between being close and being distant in romantic relationships, which can be found in many people. Since this process takes place unconsciously and compulsively, it is not surprising that it can lead to all sorts of problems and dramas. And precisely these problems and this basic life drama are made conscious, defused and even resolved by the integration of the primordial polarity.

When you integrate Primes, you are usually immediately aware of what kind of game you have played so far in your life and in how many variations, and how you have switched from one pole to another since the time of your birth. Moreover, with the integration of the Primes, you are freed from your own deepest compulsions. You can still play the same games, but now you have the freedom to choose whether you want to. In addition, new and old problems can be solved faster and you can easily recognize the problem circles you are caught up in. While the integration of the Primes does not solve all your problems, it solves the most profound one. However, since many other problems are also due to the effect of polarities, these can also be solved with little effort with the help of PEAT or other methods.

Zivorad M. Slavinski sometimes compares the effect of Primes integration with a book whose binding is broken. Imagine that your life's episodes, dramas and experiences would be the content of a big book, - the book of your life. Then the Primes or primordial polarity would form the cover of this book, and its title would indicate your most fundamental life theme, which then dramatizes itself into 1000 variations in the individual chapters of the book of your life. The integration of the Primes could then be compared to breaking the cover of the book, so that the entire binding and thus all pages of the book would begin to loosen. As a result, it would be easy to pull out the individual pages, and I can confirm from my experience that all spiritual and therapeutic efforts have a noticeably greater effect after the Primes integration and they also lead to the desired results much faster than before.

A Deep PEAT session for Primes integration typically lasts 60 to 90 minutes, which includes half an hour being spent on preparation and rework. Since it is not possible to do the Primes integration on one's own, one always needs a partner for it, one who is well trained in leading the method.

Since the time PEAT was discovered, the Primes of several thousand people around the world have been integrated, and the resultant changes were often profound, persistent and life-changing. There can only be one primordial polarity for each person. It is not necessary to integrate it more than once. If you do not want to integrate Primes or have already integrated them, you can also use the deep PEAT process independently to address and resolve other problems and psychological issues. In this case, you take any subjective problem and apply the process to it. Typically, the problem is solved within 20 to 60 minutes, depending on the severity of the problem and whether other people are involved in the problem or not.

Complex problems such as addictions or personality disorders of course need far more than just one session.

Deep PEAT and Spirituality

In his book »Peak States of Consciousness«, Grant McFetridge writes: »Although a great many people have looked for ways and means of obtaining so-called peak experiences without problematic side effects, there are still very few effective methods that are also quickly effective. In contrast to other processes that induce peak experiences, the PEAT process not only produces fast, elegant and radical results, but also works with most of the people who use it.«

As I mentioned earlier, at the end of successful Primes integration, one experiences a state beyond polarities. In this state one touches the basic unity of all beings, which many have found to be immensely beneficial and liberating.

And now the truly amazing thing: just as Grant McFetridge has claimed, almost anyone who is able to follow the steps of the deep PEAT process can access a peak state of consciousness anytime he wants to. The deep PEAT process can even trigger an awakening experience, depending on the spiritual experience or spiritual predisposition. And to my knowledge this is not possible with any other available technology in such an incredibly short time!

Further, for those who continue using the PEAT processes, they typically find that they live in steadier states of being with decreased reactivity, increased compassion and increased present-focused attention – all hallmarks of spiritual well-being.

Literature

Fitch, J., DiGirolamo, J. A., Schmuldt, L.M. (2011)
The efficacy of PEAT to address public speaking anxiety
In Energy Psychology 3, 2, November 2011

Slavinski, Z.M. (2009)
Return to oneness
http://www.vladimirstojakovic.com/store.html

Slavinski, Z.M. (2010)
Transcendence
http://www.vladimirstojakovic.com/store.html

Slavinski, Z.M. (2011)
PEAT – new pathways
http://www.vladimirstojakovic.com/store.html

http://www.eft-berlin.de/service_buecher.htm

https://www.eft-info.com/text-bibliothek/eft--forschung

http://www.eftuniverse.com/research-studies/eft-research

https://de.wikipedia.org/wiki/Klopfakupressur

About the author:

Michael Hoffmann studied psychology at the University of Salzburg, completed various training courses in the field of psychotherapy and is now specialized in the treatment of addiction disorders and traumatic diseases.

His particular passion are the work with energy psychology and especially the methods of Zivorad M. Slavinski, under whose personal training he became a PEAT trainer and coach of several other of his systems.

Michael Hoffmann lives in Munich, Germany and works in an addiction counseling Center and in his own psychotherapeutic practice. He offers workshops for PEAT and other psycho-energetic methods of Zivorad Slavinski.

Contact:
Homepage: www.peatworld.de
E-Mail: info@peatworld.de